Ultimate Bloat Buster: Your 7 Day Guide to Good Gut Health

Introduction

If you're reading this, chances are you're tired of feeling uncomfortable in your own body – the bloating, the unpredictability, the way food can sometimes feel like the enemy. Feeling like the more you try to eat, healthy, the worse you feel.

I get it. As a long-term sufferer of food intolerances myself, I've been exactly where you are.

Sixteen years ago, I could sleep 12 hours and still wake up exhausted. I ate "healthy," but I was always hungry, constantly anxious, and battling symptoms that no doctor could explain.

It wasn't until I discovered my own food intolerances and repaired my gut that everything changed – my energy returned, my focus sharpened, and I finally felt in control of my body again.

Over the past 14 years in clinical practice, I've helped thousands of people with the same struggles – bloating, fatigue, itchy skin, IBS, brain fog.

And time and again, I've seen the evidence that when you give the gut the right support, the change can be fast and powerful.

That's exactly what this 7-day reset is designed to do. In the pages ahead, you'll find practical steps, simple swaps, and strategies that actually fit into a busy life. No extremes, no gimmicks – just real changes you can feel within a week.

You're not broken. You're not imagining it. And you don't have to keep struggling. Let's get started.

Over the next seven days, I'll guide you through a step-by-step approach to identify and manage your food intolerances effectively. You'll learn practical strategies and techniques to alleviate bloating, expand your dietary choices, and regain control of your health.

And for those of you who want a little more - consider joining the full mini course. Access the Ultimate Bloat Buster 7 Day Gut Reset at https://tinyurl.com/FIAReset.

Here's what to expect - your 7 day overview.

Day 1: Understanding Food Intolerances

On Day 1, we'll dive into the world of food intolerances. We'll explore what they are, how they differ from allergies, and why they can cause digestive distress. Gain a deeper understanding of the symptoms and triggers associated with food intolerances, setting the foundation for the rest of the course.

Day 2: Identifying Your Trigger Foods

Day 2 is all about identifying your trigger foods. Discover various methods to pinpoint the specific foods that may be causing your symptoms. From elimination diets to journaling, we'll provide you with practical tools to uncover your personal triggers.

Day 3: Creating a Gut-Friendly Meal Plan

Now that you know your trigger foods, it's time to create a gut-friendly meal plan. On Day 3, we'll guide you through the process of crafting a balanced and nourishing meal plan that excludes your trigger foods while still providing all the essential nutrients your body needs.

Day 4: Managing Bloating and Digestive Discomfort

Bloating and digestive discomfort are common symptoms of food intolerances. On Day 4, we'll share effective strategies to manage these symptoms and restore comfort to your digestive system. From natural remedies to lifestyle adjustments, you'll learn practical techniques to find relief.

Day 5: Incorporating Gut-Healing Foods

Day 5 focuses on incorporating gut-healing foods into your diet. Explore a variety of foods that promote gut health and support your body's natural healing processes. We'll provide you with easy-to-follow recipes and suggestions for adding these beneficial foods to your meals.

Day 6: Mindful Eating for Gut Health

Mindful eating plays a crucial role in improving gut health. On Day 6, we'll explore the concept of mindful eating and its impact on digestion. Learn how to slow down, listen to your body's cues, and cultivate a healthier relationship with food for optimal gut function.

Day 7: Sustaining Gut Freedom

Congratulations! You've reached Day 7, where we'll discuss sustaining gut freedom beyond this mini course. Discover practical tips and strategies for maintaining a healthy and balanced lifestyle, even after the seven days are over. We'll equip you with the tools to continue your journey toward gut freedom.

Let's get started

I'm so excited that you decided to embark on this journey. You're about to discover exactly how easy it can be to build a stronger, healthier gut that is resilient, strong and less reactive - for more food freedom.

Remember, this mini course serves as a foundation for our comprehensive 12-week program, "The Food Intolerance Solution: 12 Steps to Freedom from Intolerance." If you're ready to dive deeper and experience long-term gut freedom, we invite you to explore the full program.

To learn more, visit www.foodintoleranceaustralia.com . Break free from the limitations of food intolerances through good gut health!

Day 1: Understanding Food Intolerances

Welcome to Day 1 of the Ultimate Bloat Buster: Your 7 Day Guide to Good Gut Health! Today, we'll dig into what food intolerances actually are, how they differ from allergies, and why they can cause so much discomfort. This is the foundation – and trust me, once you really understand it, things start to click.

What Are Food Intolerances?

Food intolerances happen when your body struggles to process certain foods. Unlike allergies, which involve a strong and immediate immune response, intolerances often stem from things like:

Enzyme deficiencies (e.g. lactose intolerance) Gut microbiome imbalances, Sensitivities to natural food chemicals (like histamine or salicylates) or even nutritional deficiencies.

The type I see most in clinic, and personally experienced myself, is IgG-mediated intolerance – sometimes called a "Type 3" reaction. These reactions aren't life-threatening, but they can make daily life miserable.

Food intolerance exists on a spectrum. For some, symptoms are mild and come and go. For others, the impact is significant – affecting digestion, energy, mood, and even skin.

Common symptoms include:

- Bloating,
- gas, or abdominal pain
- Diarrhoea or constipation
- Irritable bowel-type symptoms
- Nausea and fatigue
- Brain fog or poor concentration

How Are Food Intolerances Different from Allergies?

This part is important. Food allergies and food intolerances share some symptoms, but the way they behave is very different.

- **Allergies:** trigger a fast, immune-driven response. Symptoms can include hives, swelling, difficulty breathing, and in severe cases, anaphylaxis. Even tiny amounts can be dangerous – life-long avoidance is essential.

- **Intolerances:** are less severe and your management plan is more flexible. They're often dose-dependent, meaning you might tolerate small amounts but react when you eat more. Symptoms build over time rather than appearing instantly. Your gut health largely determines the strength of your reaction.

In a nutshell: Someone with an allergy may be triggered by minute exposure through cross-contamination, while someone with a food intolerance might feel fine with a small bite, but experience symptoms if they eat a whole serve.

The Gut Connection

Here's where things get interesting. Intolerances and gut health are a two-way street. If your gut is already inflamed, lacking digestive enzymes, or low in nutrients you'll likely react more strongly to certain foods.

And every reaction increases inflammation, which worsens the cycle. That's why supporting good gut health is as important as finding your trigger foods.

Your First Step

Today's action: Keep a food diary – jot down what you eat and how you feel afterwards. It doesn't need to be a big task, just capture the basics: what you ate and how you felt/how your symptoms changed. The patterns might surprise you.

In Day 2, we'll explore how to identify your personal trigger foods with practical tools like elimination diets, intolerance testing, and professional guidance.

For now, remember this: Food intolerances don't have to control your life. By understanding what's really happening in your body, you've already taken the first step toward good gut health, and freedom from intolerance.

Day 2: Identifying Your Trigger Foods

Welcome to day 2. Yesterday we talked about what food intolerances are and how they differ from allergies. Today we're diving into the practical part: figuring out which foods are causing trouble for you.

When I was first unravelling my own food sensitivities, I felt like I was playing a never-ending guessing game. One day I'd be fine with sourdough, the next I'd be so bloated/tired/sneezy I couldn't think straight.

Many of my patients come in feeling the same – confused, overwhelmed, and unsure where to start.

The reason is that trigger foods are rarely obvious. Sometimes it's not the food itself, but the combination of foods, your stress level that day, or the health of your gut lining. That's why a structured approach makes all the difference.

Tools to identify triggers

Here are the three main ways we uncover problem foods:

1: Keeping a Food & Symptom Diary

Keep a simple journal for a week. Note what you eat, when you eat it, and how you feel afterwards. Don't overthink it – even quick notes like "oats for breakfast 7am – bloated by 10am" can be revealing.

2: Elimination Diet & Rechallenge

This involves removing likely culprits (think gluten, dairy, processed foods, high-FODMAPs) for a set period, then carefully reintroducing them one at a time to see what sparks symptoms. This step takes patience, but it remains one of the most widely used tools by practitioners

How to do it

Start by eliminating the most common culprits linked to your suspected intolerance. For example: If you suspect lactose intolerance, you could switch to lactose-free dairy, choose naturally low-lactose products (the FODMAP app from Monash University can help with this), or simply avoid all dairy to keep things simple.

Keep a record of any changes in your symptoms during the elimination period. After 2–3 weeks, begin reintroducing one food group at a time and track how your body responds.

The limitations

This method isn't perfect. Many people react to more than one food group or have highly sensitive systems. That can leave them stuck in the elimination phase for months, unable to reintroduce foods successfully.

I'll admit, this was the exact experience that shifted my own approach.

Early in my career, I worked with a patient who reacted so strongly to every reintroduction that the process became almost cruel. I eventually recommended a food intolerance test.

Within weeks, we had a clear action plan and knew exactly which foods to remove to support her recovery. Her health improved, she regained lost weight, and to her joy, she fell pregnant after years of trying. From that moment on, I was sold. Testing plus personalised advice gave her hope and results in a way elimination alone never could.

A quick note of caution

If you have specific health concerns, or if you're currently pregnant or breastfeeding, an elimination diet may not be the right choice for you. In these cases, I recommend working closely with a healthcare professional or Clinical Nutritionist to make sure your diet stays balanced and nourishing throughout the process.

3: Food Sensitivity Tests

Food intolerance testing takes the guesswork out of the process. Instead of spending weeks trying to piece together your trigger foods through elimination, testing can provide a clear snapshot of what your body is reacting to.

How it works

A small blood sample (which can be done with a simple finger-prick at home) is analysed for reactions to hundreds of foods.

The results show you which foods your immune system is reacting to most strongly, helping to identify the culprits quickly and clearly.

Why it helps

The biggest advantage of testing is specificity.
You're not cutting out whole food groups
"just in case." You can focus on exactly what
needs to go, while keeping as much variety
and enjoyment in your diet as possible.

Thinking back to my patient mentioned
before - this was the game changer for her.
She was terrified to add anything back in
because every trial re-triggered her
symptoms. Once we did a food intolerance
test, we discovered just a few strong
offenders she needed to avoid.

If you decide to go down the path of testing (or are reading this whilst awaiting your test results) you're on the fast track to finding your personalised approach. Your results will show us exactly what foods to avoid and what we can challenge to find the cause of your symptoms.

Things to keep in mind

Food intolerance testing is a powerful tool, but it's not a stand-alone solution. Test results need to be interpreted in the context of your symptoms, medical history, and gut health as a whole. That's why I always recommend pairing test results with a consultation – so you're not just left with a long list of foods to avoid, but with a clear roadmap for recovery.

Disclaimer:

If you've tried journaling, elimination diets, or even testing and still feel stuck, it might be time for extra support. Working with a Clinical Nutritionist or Dietitian who understands food intolerances can save you months of trial and error.

I've seen patients come in with diets reduced to fewer than 10 foods because they were afraid of reacting. With personalised support, we expanded their options, reduced symptoms, and rebuilt their trust in food. The real win isn't just fewer symptoms but the freedom to enjoy food and life again.

Note: Though we focus largely on serving our Australian community at Food Intolerance Australia, we offer telehealth consultations to patients world-wide. Reach out for support any time - www.foodintoleranceaustralia.com

Day 3: Creating a Gut-Friendly Meal Plan

By now, you've likely got the picture that food intolerances aren't an isolated issue. They're closely tied to the state of your gut. A healthy gut helps you digest and absorb food, regulate your immune system, and even balance mood and energy. When your gut is out of balance, intolerances often flare.

Your gut works hard every day. It breaks food down into usable nutrients, produces the enzymes and acids needed for digestion, and houses trillions of microbes that protect you from harmful bacteria. It even communicates directly with your brain, influencing mood, focus, and stress resilience.

When your gut is out of balance, you feel it. I often see patients who think they've suddenly developed new intolerances, when in fact it's just that their gut balance has shifted.

A round of antibiotics, a stressful period at work, a patch of uber eats-ing and wine-ing a little too often, or even poor sleep can reduce capacity for your digestive system to do its daily work and healing. Our perceivable symptom - foods we once tolerated are suddenly problematic.

The encouraging part is that gut health is dynamic, which means it can be repaired. When you bring back balance through better food choices, key nutrients, and supportive lifestyle habits, tolerance often improves and symptoms start to fade.

Why Meal Planning is Helpful:

Meal planning can have a huge impact on your ability to heal your gut. powerful. It doesn't need to be complicated, a little structure goes a long way. The goal is to help you make choices that strengthen your gut rather than stress it. Planning ahead also takes the pressure off busy days, reduces reliance on processed "quick fixes," and ensures you're consistently feeding your body what it needs to repair.

Meal Planning Guidelines:

1. Identify Trigger Foods:Refer back to your list of trigger foods and make sure to avoid them when planning your meals. If you've had a food intolerance test with us, you'll see a list of substitute foods right next to each substitute food in your report.

2. **Focus on Whole Foods**: Centre meals around quality protein, add colourful vegetables, then include gut-friendly extras like fermented foods, healthy fats, or a small serve of whole grains if tolerated.

3. **Include Gut-Friendly Ingredients:**Incorporate gut-friendly ingredients like probiotic-rich foods (yogurt, kefir), fibre-rich foods (fruits, vegetables, legumes – if tolerated), and anti-inflammatory foods (turmeric, ginger, garlic, extra virgin olive oil, salmon etc).

4. **Rotate your foods:** Don't eat the same thing every day. Variety feeds different "good bugs" in your gut and helps build resilience. Variety can also help prevent forming new intolerances.

5. **Experiment with Cooking Methods:**Try different cooking methods to find what works best for you. If your digestion is particularly sensitive right now, you might find slow-cooked meats, poached fish, and simply steamed vegetables are the most soothing.

6. **Tips:** If bloating and constipation are ongoing issues, blending can help too. A daily blended option, like a chicken-and-veg soup cooked slow and pureed smooth, can help ease constipation and bloating.

7. **Prep in Advance:** When eating out, be sure to review menus in advance and/or call ahead to ask for their allergens list. Try to plan your meal ahead of time - also look at the sides and don't be afraid to call and ask if menu items can be altered. Tip: If a restaurant is willing to alter a meal to accommodate your dietary needs it's a good sign that they are preparing the meals fresh. Don't be afraid to ask!

8. **Plan for balance:** Remember, your goal is to support repair, not restrict unnecessarily. Don't be hard on yourself if you 'slip up' - just try to be as consistent as you can when it's within your control. The end goal is to not rely on restriction - this is just a temporary step to help optimise the healing and provide symptom relief.

Gut-Friendly Recipe Suggestions:

Gut-Calm Omelette

When you want something quick that keeps you satisfied.

- 2 eggs
- Handful baby spinach
- 1 zucchini, grated
- Handful mushrooms, chopped
- 1 tsp ground turmeric
- Sprinkle pumpkin seeds
- Olive oil for cooking
- ¼ avocado, sliced
- Squeeze of fresh lemon juice

Instructions: Sauté zucchini and mushrooms in olive oil. Add spinach, then pour over whisked eggs with turmeric. Cook gently until set, top with avocado slices and lemon juice. Sprinkle with pumpkin seeds before serving.

Benefits:

- Eggs + seeds: rich in zinc, vital for gut repair
- Avocado + olive oil: healthy fats that calm inflammation
- Zucchini, mushrooms + avo: fibre for microbial balance
- Lemon juice: vitamin C for collagen + bitters to aid protein and fat digestion
- Turmeric: soothing, anti-inflammatory, and supports serotonin

Soothing Green Smoothie

For when you need something gentle and refreshing.

Ingredients:

- 1 cup baby spinach
- ½ frozen zucchini
- ½ cup pineapple or papaya
- 1 tbsp chia seeds
- 1 cup unsweetened coconut milk

Benefits:

- Spinach and zucchini provide fibre to feed healthy microbes.
- Pineapple and papaya contain enzymes that support digestion and reduce inflammation.
- Chia seeds help with regularity, are a great source of insoluble fibre - which acts as a broom that sweeps the gut clean, and provide anti-inflammatory fats.

Comforting Chicken + Veg Soup

A blended option for sensitive tummies.

- 1 Chicken breast, poached

- 2 carrots, chopped

- 1 zucchini, chopped

- 1 cup spinach

- 1 clove garlic (if tolerated)

- 4 cups bone broth

Simmer until vegetables are soft. Blend until smooth.

Benefits: Poached chicken is easy to digest and provides protein for repair. Garlic adds antimicrobial support. Blending eases bloating & constipation.

Anti-Bloat Salmon Bowl

Simple dinner with big gut health pay-off.

- 1 fillet salmon, baked or poached
- ½ cup quinoa or basmati rice
- Steamed broccoli + zucchini
- Handful of rocket
- Drizzle of olive oil + Squeeze of lemon

Benefits: Salmon provides anti-inflammatory omega-3s. Quinoa offers zinc, protein and fibre without the heaviness of wheat or use basmati for a lighter option (rinse well to reduce starch and soak lightly to support easy digestion). Broccoli supports detox and gut repair. Lemon juice aids fat digestion.

Reset Lentil + Veg Stew

Hearty yet gentle on digestion.

- 1 cup red lentils (soaked + rinsed well)
- 1 zucchini, diced
- 1 carrot, diced
- 1 stick celery
- 1 tsp cumin + coriander powder
- 4 cups veg stock
- Simmer until soft.

Benefits: Red lentils are easier to digest than other legumes. Spices add antimicrobial support. Carrot + celery provide fibre to feed microbes.

Nourish Bowl with Turkey + Avocado

Perfect for lunch on the go.

- 100g cooked turkey breast (sliced)
- Steamed green beans
- 1/2 an avocado
- Handful leafy greens
- Sprinkle sesame seeds
- Dressing olive oil + cider vinegar or lemon juice

Benefits: Turkey is a lean, zinc-rich protein. Avocado soothes inflammation. Sesame seeds provide calcium + healthy fats.

When planning your meals, there are a few key tips to keep in mind – things like learning how to read labels, planning snacks in advance, and building a support network.

1. Read Labels and Ingredient Lists

When you're living with food intolerances, it's important to build a habit of reading labels. Ingredient lists often hide unexpected triggers, from additives to small amounts of gluten, lactose, or fructose.

Get familiar with the different names your trigger foods can hide under. For example, lactose might show up as whey, curd, or milk solids.

Knowing these terms means you can make confident choices and avoid accidental slip-ups.

Hot tip: unless you have an **allergy** or coeliac disease, "may contain traces of…" should not mean the food is unsafe for you. That warning is there for those who can react to even microscopic amounts via cross-contamination, not for those with intolerances.

Having food intolerances doesn't mean missing out. There are so many alternatives now that make it easier to enjoy a wide variety of meals. If you can't tolerate lactose or dairy, try almond, coconut, or oat milk.

If gluten is an issue, swap for rice, quinoa, or gluten-free flours.

Don't be afraid to experiment. Trying new substitutes and recipes not only keeps meals interesting, it helps you discover options you actually enjoy.

Variety is a big part of keeping your gut (and your taste buds) happy. Communicate Your Needs Eating out or heading to a social event can feel stressful, but clear communication makes a huge difference.

Let friends, family, or restaurant staff know about your intolerances so they can help you find safe options. It's not about being difficult – it's about protecting your health.

Asking how a meal is prepared or checking ingredients before you order can prevent setbacks and give you peace of mind.

Build a Support Network

Managing food intolerances can feel isolating at times, but you don't have to do it alone. Lean on supportive friends and family, and connect with others who've been through similar challenges. Online communities, local groups, or even fellow patients can share tips and encouragement. Having people who "get it" not only provides practical advice, it also helps you feel seen and understood – which makes the journey much easier.

Tomorrow, we will discuss simple and effective ways to reduce bloating and discomfort.

Day 4: Managing Bloating and Discomfort

So, by now you've probably noticed a pattern. Bloating isn't only about overeating or "bad" trigger foods – it's often about the state of your gut.

Inflammation makes your digestive system more sensitive, so even simple foods can leave you puffed up and uncomfortable. I see this in clinic all the time. Patients say, "I bloat no matter what I eat" or "The healthier I eat, the worse I feel."

After 14 years in practice, working with thousands of patients, I can tell you the problem is rarely the food itself. It's usually an inflamed, reactive gut environment creating food sensitivity. Once that inflammation is soothed, the very same foods often cause far fewer issues.

Why bloating and inflammation are linked

When your gut lining is irritated or your microbes are out of balance, food ferments where it shouldn't. Gas builds up. Transit slows. And suddenly you feel heavy, swollen, and on edge. Calm the inflammation, and digestion runs smoother, gas production drops, and bloating finally eases.

Your Gut-Calming Toolkit

Here are some of the strategies I use myself
and with patients:

- Slow down meals – chew well, pause
  between bites, avoid eating on the run.
- Cook foods gently – steaming, stewing,
  or poaching makes foods easier to
  digest.
- Choose anti-inflammatory staples –
  think turmeric, ginger, oily fish, olive oil,
  leafy greens.
- Hydrate smartly – sip water through the
  day and avoid large drinks with meals.
- Move lightly after eating – a gentle walk
  or stretching supports digestion.
- Calm your nervous system – stress fuels
  inflammation, so try a few deep breaths
  prior to eating each meal.

Lessons learned in clinic: One of my early patients came in convinced she was "allergic to everything." Her bloating was so severe she had cut back to fewer than ten "safe" foods. She was hesitant but agreed to a gut health check - here we found significant imbalances and clear signs of inflammation. Instead of removing more foods, we focused on calming her gut first: slow-cooked meals, targeted supplements, and soothing stress support. Within weeks her bloating eased, her food list expanded, and her confidence grew. That's the power of treating the underlying issue, not just relying on eliminating foods.

Today's Action: Pick One Calming Strategy

So, now you know bloating isn't just about the food - it's about the state of your gut. Inflammation, stress, and poor digestion can all make simple meals feel like the enemy. Today, pick just one of the following strategies to practise:

- Mindful eating – slow down, chew well, and take breaks between bites.
- Gentle movement – a 10–15 min walk after meals or child's pose if you're gassy.
- Soothing tea – peppermint or ginger before or after meals.

Track it: Jot down how you felt before and after the meal. Did your belly feel lighter? Less pressure? More comfortable? Keep it simple. Focus on one action today and notice the shift. Tomorrow we'll build on this.

Day 5: Incorporating Gut-Healing Foods

I've mentioned my own personal journey with food sensitivity - like most I thought cutting things out was the only answer. And it really helped - at first. My energy soared, my mood improved and I lost 7 kgs in a few weeks with only minor tweaks to my diet.

However, while I felt great, I also understood that my diet was likely unsustainable long term. As a 3rd year student of clinical nutrition, I was pretty passionate about following a healthy diet, but I also knew this level of restriction would become difficult - I had to find another way.

I began researching and experimenting methods of actually repairing my gut and reducing my sensitivity.

I focused on mindful eating, correcting posture while eating, optimising my portions, balancing my meals, and layering in foods which heal, repair, support or aid the digestive system - one by one.

The changes were easy, simple and minimal - I cooked with Bone broth, swapped sourdough for gluten free bread topped with avocado, and kept snacks simple and nutritious like apple slices with natural peanut butter. I brought in colourful veggies at every meal and upped my omega-3s followed by a fresh glass of lemon water.

Within weeks my energy was incredible, my skin was constantly getting compliments, and I woke up without a headache or bloating. Over the years in clinic, I've seen the same thing: avoiding trigger foods helps, but it's gut-healing that transforms health long-term.

Quick tips for gut repair: Nutrients like zinc, vitamin A, and omega-3s repair your gut lining. Amino acids soothe irritation. Prebiotics and probiotics rebuild balance.

Here are some simple ways you can start today:

1. **Fibre-Rich Foods:**Incorporate fibre-rich foods such as fruits, vegetables, whole grains, and legumes into your meals. Fiber helps keep your digestive system regular, aids in proper bowel movements, and prevents constipation, which can contribute to bloating.

2. **Fermented Foods:**Add fermented foods like yogurt, kimchi, sauerkraut, and kefir to your diet. These foods are rich in probiotics, which help balance the gut microbiome, improve digestion, and reduce bloating.

3. **Ginger and Turmeric:** Incorporate ginger and turmeric into your meals or enjoy them as teas. These spices have anti-inflammatory properties that can help soothe the gut, reduce inflammation, and relieve bloating.

4. **Bone Broth:** Consider adding bone broth to your diet. It is rich in collagen and amino acids that support gut lining health, reduce inflammation, and aid in digestion.

5. **Omega-3 Fatty Acids:**Include sources of omega-3 fatty acids like fatty fish (salmon, sardines) or chia seeds in your meals. Omega-3s help reduce inflammation in the gut and promote a healthy digestive system.

6. **Peppermint:** Enjoy peppermint tea or incorporate fresh peppermint leaves into your meals. Peppermint has been shown to relax the muscles of the gastrointestinal tract, relieving bloating and discomfort.

7. **Bitter foods:**Beautiful Bitters for Good Gut Health: Introducing foods such as bitter greens, herbs, and certain fruits, offer unique properties that support digestive health and alleviate bloating. Bitters are so effective they deserve a full page write up. Read on to find out more.

8. **Zinc rich foods:** Oysters are the richest natural source of zinc, followed by other animal foods such as beef, lamb, pork, chicken thighs and legs, turkey dark meat, liver, sardines, mackerel, salmon and eggs. Plant-based options include pumpkin seeds, sunflower seeds, hemp seeds, sesame seeds (tahini), cashews, almonds, chickpeas, lentils, quinoa and oats.

9. **Vitamin A:** Include liver, cod liver oil, egg yolks, full-fat dairy (if tolerated), and oily fish like salmon and mackerel. Plant-based sources provide beta-carotene which the body converts into vitamin A, including carrots, sweet potato, pumpkin, butternut squash, capsicum, spinach, kale and other leafy greens.

10. **Amino acids that soothe the gut:**
Glutamine-rich foods such as bone broth, chicken, turkey, beef, fish, eggs, cabbage, spinach, parsley and beets. Glycine, another gut-soothing amino acid, is abundant in gelatin, bone broth, pork skin, chicken skin, and cuts of meat cooked on the bone.

Bitter foods and why to use them

1. **Bitter Greens:** Embrace leafy greens like kale, rocket, spinach. These nutrient-dense greens are packed with fibre, vitamins, and minerals that promote a healthy gut. The bitterness stimulates digestive enzymes, supporting digestion and reducing bloating.

2. **Fresh Herbs:** Experiment with fresh herbs like parsley, coriander, mint. Their natural bitterness not only adds flavour to your dishes but also stimulates the production of digestive juices, helping to break down food and prevent bloating.

3. **Citrus Fruits:** Citrus fruits like grapefruits, lemons, oranges possess a pleasant bitterness. They are rich in vitamin C & antioxidants to support gut health.

4. **Dark Chocolate:** Indulge in a square or two of dark chocolate with a high cocoa percentage. The bitterness of dark chocolate stimulates the production of digestive enzymes and encourages healthy gut function.

As always, listen to your body and make changes gradually. Everyone's gut responds differently, so try these gut-healing foods and notice what feels best for you. Tomorrow, we'll dive into mindful eating and how it can make digestion calmer and easier. Step by step, you're building the foundations for a gut that works with you, not against you.

Day 6: Mindful Eating for Good Gut Health

If mindful eating seems impossible– I get it! As a busy working mum of two, running two businesses and constantly feeling time-poor, there are plenty of times I've eaten on the run or while distracted. It does take conscious effort to eat mindfully - but the pay off is worth it.

I used to eat most meals in a hurry. Breakfast on the way, lunch at my desk, dinner while working or researching. I thought I was being efficient, but all I really did was leave my gut in chaos. I'd finish a meal and immediately feel bloated, foggy, I was constantly hungry and running on adrenaline.

Through my studies and clinical work I realised how much difference mindful eating makes. I now begin with a few breaths before meals, putting my fork down between bites, and actually tasting my food. The benefit is huge – digestion calms, you feel satisfied from less food, and the bloating eases quickly.

From a clinical perspective, this makes perfect sense. When you're stressed, rushing, or distracted, your body stays in "fight or flight" mode. In this state, digestion is suppressed – stomach acid drops, enzymes are reduced, motility slows. But when you activate "rest and digest" by slowing down, chewing properly, and eating without distractions, your body can break down food properly and absorb nutrients more effectively. Not to mention enjoying it more!

Let's discuss the benefits of mindful eating:

1. **Enhanced Digestive Enzyme Production:** When you eat mindfully, you engage all your senses and thoroughly chew your food, allowing the release of saliva and digestive enzymes in your mouth. These enzymes aid in breaking down food more effectively, supporting optimal digestion and nutrient absorption.

2. **Improved Recognition of Food Reactions:** You become more attuned to how different foods make you feel. You start recognising any adverse reactions or sensitivities, such as bloating, gas, or discomfort. This empowers you to make informed choices about your diet and avoid triggers that may negatively impact your gut health.

3. **Reduced Stress on the Digestive System:** Mindful eating promotes relaxation during meals. By taking your time, enjoying your meal without distractions, you allow your body to enter a rest-and-digest mode. This reduces stress on the digestive system, improves nutrient absorption, and minimises the likelihood of bloating or indigestion.

4. **Mind-Gut Connection:** When you slow down and bring calm to your meals, you're not just eating – you're sending signals of safety to your digestive system. This shift helps reduce stress-driven gut issues like IBS or indigestion, and over time, builds a healthier, happier gut. You'll also begin loving this down time and will feel calmer, clearer and more focused - you'll be addicted to othis practice in no time!

Making Mindful Eating Easy:

- **Take your time:** Eat slowly, chew thoroughly, and savour the flavours.

- **Eliminate distractions:** Minimise distractions like phones, TV, or work during meals to focus solely on the eating experience.

- **Tune into hunger and fullness cues:** Pay attention to your body's signals of hunger and fullness to guide your eating patterns.

- **Express gratitude:** Take a moment to appreciate the ability to take time out and enjoy your food.

- **Practice good posture and breathe:** Sit up straight, breathe and relax. This can help minimise indigestion and bloating and also helps you to not rush meals.

- **Consider setting a timer:** This may sound funny, but setting a timer for 5-15 minutes to eat without distractions can work wonderfully for busy-bees who struggle to find the time to relax. Setting the timer allows you to switch off - everything can wait 5 minutes. Knowing the timer will ring prevents the need to check the time - which prevents accidental distractions and stressors. If you're always on the go, I strongly recommend this option.

Making space for mindful eating each day can make a real difference to your gut. Slowing down helps you tune in to your body, spot food reactions earlier, and take pressure off your digestive system. Tomorrow we'll pull everything together and talk about how to keep your gut in good shape well beyond this 7-day reset. You're doing brilliantly – stay with it, the best is yet to come.

Day 7: Beyond the Reset

You've made it to Day 7 – well done! By now you've seen how small, consistent changes can ease bloating, calm your gut, and give you more energy. The real secret though? This isn't the finish line. It's the starting point.

Gut health is a moving target. Stress, sleep, food choices, and even life seasons will shift what your body needs. The key is learning how to check in with yourself, listen to your signals, and make steady adjustments over time.

Think of the last week as your reset button. You've pressed pause on the cycle of symptoms and overwhelm, and created space for healing to begin.

The next step is about building on these foundations – expanding your food variety, strengthening your microbiome, and supporting long-term resilience.

The good news? You don't have to do it alone. That's exactly why I created Food Intolerance Australia testing packages, consultations, and extra resources. Testing helps pinpoint hidden triggers, and from there we can map out a simple, practical plan that works for you.

👉 If you're ready for the next step, book your test or consultation today and let's keep your momentum going.
www.foodintoleranceaustralia.com/testing

✨ Remember: gut health freedom isn't about perfection. It's about consistency, curiosity, and knowing your body better than ever. You've already started. Now keep going.

Personal note: When I first started this journey myself, I didn't know how powerful simple, consistent habits could be. But over time I saw it in my own health, and later in my patients: Gut health isn't transformed overnight. It's built, day by day, with food, rest, and self-awareness.

This week has given you tools to start:

- Understanding the role of food intolerances and gut imbalances
- Identifying your own food triggers and patterns Using strategies to calm bloating and inflammation
- Adding gut-healing foods to your plate
- Practising mindful eating so your gut feels supported

Where to From Here?

You've just completed the Ultimate Bloat Buster Reset – that alone is worth celebrating.

If you've noticed even small changes – less bloating, calmer digestion, a little more energy – take that as proof your body responds when given the right support.

The next step is simple: keep building. Testing and consultation provide clarity, while your daily habits create lasting results.

If you're ready, book your test at www.foodintoleranceaustralia.com and let's map out a plan that works for you.

Prefer more structure and accountability? Join the 7 day mini course at https://tinyurl.com/FIAReset, where I guide you step by step with extra tips, games, and checklists to help these habits stick.

Most importantly, remember gut health isn't about perfection – it's about consistency and listening to your body.

Small steps compound into big wins. You've already started. Now keep going.

✦ Here's to calmer digestion, steadier energy, and more food freedom.

Thank you for reading Ultimate Bloat Buster: Your 7 day guide to good gut health, I sincerely hope you got a lot out of it. I loved sharing this journey with you. If you'd like to learn more, here are some ways to connect:

- Follow us on instagram
  @FoodIntoleranceAustralia
- Watch my youtube channel
  at https://www.youtube.com/@Jennifer
  MayFIA

- Join the Ultimate Bloat Buster 7 Day Gut
  Reset at: https://tinyurl.com/FIAReset

Here's to you and your health. I hope this guide has inspired you to take small, daily actions that support good gut health for life.

Remember, you don't have to figure it all out on your own. My team and I are always here to help. Reach out any time: info@foodintoleranceaustralia.com

To your health,

Jennifer May

Clinical Nutritionist / Speaker/ Author

Director, Food Intolerance Australia